Lupus the Wolf

Lupus the Wolf

Fifty-Nine Years With Thomas and Lupus

TWILA J. MCKAY-SMITH

-Smith was born in Topeka, Kansas, to Mary and Richard McKay. She and her husband, Thomas, have a daughter, son, granddaughter, two grandsons, two great-grandsons, and one great-granddaughter.

She and Thom reside in Florida, enjoying the weather and each other. In Twila's spare time, she crochets, reads, and works in her church and community.

ISBN: 1537662074
ISBN 13: 9781537662077

Library of Congress Control Number: 2016915489
CreateSpace Independent Publishing Platform
North Charleston, South Carolina

To Thomas Smith Jr.

Praise ye the Lord, O give thanks unto the Lord, for he is good for his mercy endureth forever. Who can utter the mighty acts of the Lord? Who can shew forth all His praise? (Psalm 106:1–2)

Praise ye the Lord. Praise the Lord, O my soul. While I live will I praise the Lord: I will sing praises unto my God while I have being. (Psalm 146:1–2)

Every good gift and every perfect gift is from above, and cometh down from the Father of lights, there is no variableness, neither shadow of turning. (James 1:17)

CONTENTS

INTRODUCTION

This is my story of faith, hope, and love. It was a beautiful morning in Tampa, Florida, and as I was walking around the base, I prayed to the Lord. Thom was having a lupus flare that had been attacking his body for a couple of weeks. I was at peace, watching the beautiful birds in the area and looking out at the water as the ships went out to sea, knowing the Lord was with us.

It was then that the Lord put the idea in my mind to write about Thom's illness and how I have coped during his flares. Everything I went through before marrying Thom prepared me for a lupus ride, but I couldn't have done it without the Lord's help. It was time to share with family and friends how the Lord had brought me through it all. I pray this book will help others who are caregivers to people who are ill and inspire them to persevere through their trials.

Thom amazes me with how much pain he can take. I am a big baby and need all the medication I can get to help me withstand pain. When our kids were living at home, he was a good father, even though he was suffering daily with pain and depression.

Many people have commented, "He looks good," even when he is going through a rough time of the illness. I decided it was time to share with others what they cannot see when he is going through a flare.

■ ■ ■

I met Thomas Smith Jr. ("Lucky") in October 1955 when he was stationed at Forbes Air Force Base in Topeka, Kansas, serving our country.

We dated for one year and five months. He proposed to me in December 1956, and then on March 3, 1957, I became Mrs. Thomas Smith, Jr.

We traveled from Kansas to Elizabeth, New Jersey; Albuquerque, New Mexico (Kirkland AFB); the Philippines (Clark AFB); Middletown, Pennsylvania (Olmsted AFB); back to the Philippines (Clark AFB); and

Rome, New York (Griffiss AFB). I then lived in Salina, Kansas, with other "waiting wives," and Thom went to Thailand. The kids and I were separated from Thom for eleven months while he was stationed in Thailand. Next, we moved to Wrightstown, New Jersey (McGuire AFB); Madrid, Spain (Torrejon AFB); and Sacramento, California (Mather AFB). Then he retired from the military. In later years, after Thom's retirement, we moved to Lancaster/Palmdale, California.

While Thom was in Thailand, he collapsed at work. He was the only airplane electrician at the base, and he had to get the planes repaired so the pilots could continue their assignments. The air force sent a couple of electricians to help him during the last part of his tour. He recovered enough to perform his duties and later returned to the States for another assignment.

Thom suffered from alopecia (hair loss), shortness of breath, mouth sores, extreme tiredness, lupus fog, rashes, water around his heart, mental confusion, severe joint pain, and kidney infections, but he persevered and kept working in order to support his family. I would sometimes get upset because people kept saying, "He doesn't look sick, he looks good." I often had to remember Galatians 5:22:

> Fruits of the spirit, love, joy, peace, patience, kindness, goodness, faithfulness, gentleness, and self-control.

Lupus the Wolf

Many people have never heard of lupus, and we discovered that even many doctors are not knowledgeable about it. Facts about the disease were not publicized.

Thom went to many doctors without getting an accurate diagnosis. Some doctors called him a hypochondriac, and some said that he should find another doctor. But with faith in the Lord and prayers from friends and family, we have come far.

Lupus affects the family as well as the person who has lupus. The family sacrifices a lot, because the lupus patient is always in pain and extremely tired. Thom often did not feel like going shopping or on family outings or other activities, so I would take the kids shopping and to the park or to church or for car rides, just doing things to help them have a normal childhood despite the change in our lives.

I now know how important support groups can be in helping any chronically ill person or anyone with an autoimmune disease live a life with hope.

Lupus imitates many diseases, which Thom's doctors could not diagnose, and then it disappears until it attacks the body in some other way.

Thom began having symptoms of lupus in 1960, but the doctors did not diagnose it until 1994.

I had never heard of lupus until Thom told me that his sister had it, and then I started reading about the disease. Back then, the information available about lupus was devastating. The information stated that you did not have long to live if you had lupus.

I traveled around the world with Thom for twenty years before he retired, and I saw his struggles with low-grade fever, anxiety, lupus fog, lupus rashes, breathing problems, painful and swollen joints, water around his heart, allergies, prolonged fatigue, anemia, Raynaud's disease (numb fingers and toes), and alopecia (hair loss).

I saw that Thom was under a lot of stress because he wanted to continue his military career, but I was afraid that because he felt ill all the time, he would soon have to get out of the air force. He was so dedicated to serving his country and to taking care of his family.

It was especially hard when we traveled across the country, from state to state, because we had to travel without stopping. Being Negroes (black), we were not allowed to spend the night in a motel or hotel. But I know that the Lord was watching over us, because I was at peace wherever we went.

Why I Love Him

I wrote this letter to Thom in January 1995.

> Dear Thom,
>   After almost thirty-eight years of marriage, I still love
> you for your caring and all the sacrifices that you made

to please me. You're always thinking of what would be good for me and what I would look good in. You share the housework and are always thinking of others' feelings. That is one of your best features, because we need "more love and less paperwork," as Pearl Bailey said. You're always surprising me with little gifts when I come home from a trip. Whenever I wanted to start a new adventure, you never complained but just helped me do research and said, "Go for it." When I get on the wrong track, you steer me back in the right direction.

You show me how to shop for bargains but purchase top-quality items. We've lived all over the world, and whenever I had to leave my job to follow you, you felt bad that I had to start all over again. That's why I haven't wanted or needed anyone else—you have fulfilled all my needs.

Our life together has not been perfect, but you have so many good qualities that I don't dwell on the things that challenged us. They helped us grow and be stronger. I pray the Lord gives us thirty-eight more years together to share with our grandchildren. You have so much to teach them. You are a gentleman who opens my door, and you hold my hand as we walk down the street.

When I've been under the weather, you've always been there. When the job gets to me, you make me focus on God and what my gifts are so that I can go and do my best job, no matter how I feel.

You're my husband, consultant, and best friend. God bless you with many more years of sharing and caring for me and the family.

Love,
Your wife, Twila

1

TRAVELING WITH A FOOD BASKET

I was born and raised in Topeka, Kansas. My dad worked for the Atchison, Topeka, and Santa Fe Railway Company, and my parents' family of eight, which consisted of six children as well as my mother and my father, traveled a lot by train all over the western and central parts of the United States. Once, my dad took all six of his kids on a train trip to San Francisco, California, all by himself when we were five to thirteen years old. We traveled on the Atchison, Topeka and Santa Fe Railway, and then we transferred to the Rock Island Line in Salt Lake City, Utah. I was very happy to be with my dad; he was very compassionate and patient with us. We had a large food basket that my mom had prepared for the trip, because at that time "Negroes" could not eat in the club car or dining car.

We spent a day in Utah on the Fourth of July. We did not hear firecrackers, because Utah had fire codes during the dry season. We were used to hearing firecrackers and fireworks on the Fourth of July, so it was strange *not* to hear anything.

We arrived in Oakland, California, and caught a ferry to San Francisco. The evening was cold, and we were not prepared for the weather. It was summer, and we thought we would not need jackets, but San Francisco was chilly at night on the water.

After visiting family, meeting cousins, and seeing the city, we returned to the train station to return home. On our trip back from San Francisco, we again rode the Atchison, Topeka and Santa Fe Railway, but we returned on a different route, passing through different cities that we had not seen before.

I felt very proud of my dad and the way the conductors and attendants treated him. Because of the camaraderie they shared as fellow railroad workers, we kids were treated to ice cream and other delights.

At ten years old, I was aware of my surroundings and of how people showed their care and love toward one another.

Our family also traveled a lot to Kansas City, Missouri, and Chicago, Illinois, to visit family. These traveling experiences prepared me for the journey I would have with Thom and helped me adjust to the many moves we made during the twenty years my husband served our country. The Lord blessed me with the ability to cope and try new things.

Not a Sports Widow

As a young girl, I often sat with my dad and watched football, baseball, basketball, track, and boxing. My dad would watch a boxing match and start ducking when someone was hit. I asked him why he ducked, but he would just look at me and smile and then go back to watching the boxing match.

Because my dad had taught me all about each sport, I was not a sports widow when I married Thom. I could name all the players on the teams we watched. The Brooklyn Dodgers were my dad's favorite team, and Thom liked the New York Yankees. I now also enjoy watching college football.

2

A DYNAMIC MEETING

I met Thomas Smith Jr. in October 1955, when he was stationed at Forbes Air Force Base. Thom had seen me out the window of his barracks when I was with my sister and her boyfriend. He later said that he had wanted to jump out of the window to meet me, but he had just gotten out of the shower and didn't have any clothes on. We left before he finished dressing, so he got my phone number from a friend, who happened to be my sister's boyfriend. He called me, and I invited him to my birthday party. A month later, he attended my party, and from that point on, we went everywhere together. Thom taught me how to drive a stick shift—what a thrill!

Thom started attending New Mount Zion Baptist Church so that he could continue to date me. We dated until he proposed to me in December 1956. We were married March 3, 1957, in front of my parents' fireplace.

During the first few years of our marriage, we had one car. At first, I would drive Thom to work in the morning and then drive to town for school. I graduated from high school two months later.

It was during this time that I learned joy and patience, because I never knew when Thom would be deployed or when he would come home from work. But I had the joy of being married to him.

> My brethren, count it all joy when ye fall into divers temp-
> tations. Knowing this, that the trying of your faith wor-
> keth patience. (James 1:2–3)

I had been taught that a dutiful wife would take care of the household and be a support for her spouse. My great-aunt taught me how to drive when I was fifteen years old, and I have been driving ever since. I felt that having a relationship with the Lord and keeping my eyes on Him has helped me get through all our travels. We were frequently moving, changing jobs, and meeting new people. We also had to adjust to different types of weather over the years. I have lived through tornados, hurricanes, typhoons, humidity, blizzards, floods, and earthquakes.

3

TRAILER LIVING

We lived in a trailer on base for ten months, and during that time, I leaned on the Lord for support. I was used to a house that had plenty of room in which to move around, so living in the trailer was a big adjustment. Our trailer contained a sitting room–kitchen combination, a bedroom, and a bathroom with a shower. Our bed was against the wall, and it took a lot of patience to make the bed. Two people could not be in the kitchen at the same time. But Thom and I adjusted to the trailer, and we made it a home with our special touches.

In February 1958, I found out that I was pregnant. Thom had decided to get out of the air force and return to his hometown in New Jersey. Back then, the airlines would not let you fly after you were six months pregnant, so I flew to New Jersey early in my pregnancy and was on my own there until Thom was released from the air force. Our daughter, Collette, was born October 5, 1958, in Elizabeth General Hospital, Elizabeth, New Jersey.

Thomas spent seventy-eight days in New Jersey as a civilian. Then he decided that he wanted to serve his country and have more security for his family. Guess what? Yes, he reenlisted in the air force.

4

BEING A "NEGRO"

On December 17, 1958, we arrived at Kirkland AFB, in Albuquerque, New Mexico. We went to see several apartments that were advertised for rent, but when we arrived, we were told each time that they could not rent to us because the other renters would not like having us living above or below them. One real estate agent tried to take us to look at a large barn out in a field, and we said no before we even arrived at the barn. After that, I would always call and ask if they rented to "Negroes" before we drove to see a home.

Finally, we found a furnished duplex close to the base, but it was filthy. Thom could see that it had potential, so we decided to take it. The stove was crusty, and the refrigerator was slimy. It took us two weeks to clean up the refrigerator so that we could use it. Moreover, the couch was sagging—when you sat on it, it sounded like someone was squeezing the air out of a ball.

We asked if we could remove the furniture, which belonged to the owners, and they allowed us to store it in their barn. We then bought four rooms of furniture for about one hundred dollars. We painted the rooms and bought plastic curtains for the windows. After we had cleaned the place up, our landlady's daughter came over and said how nice it was. She asked if her mom could come over and see the place. We said yes, and the landlady came over. She exclaimed about how nice it was, and then she said, "By the way, the next month rent is going up." She stated that we could pay the increased price or move out, because she could always rent it out to someone else. We stayed because it was hard to find places what would rent to "Negroes".

Thom was an airplane electrician, so he worked out in the sun a lot. In later years, we found out that the sun was bad for some people who had lupus. He started getting extremely tired and easily upset. He also had mouth sores, and he was losing his hair. The doctors were very puzzled about his illness; they were unable to diagnose his disease.

5

CARABAO COUNTRY

A year later, on December 17, 1959, we learned that we were going to be leaving Albuquerque for a tour at Clark AFB, in the Philippines. Collette and I remained in the States until Thom found a house for us to live in.

I lived in Elizabeth with my mother-in-law, and I worked around the corner from the house in a coat factory for a few months. I also worked as a ward secretary at a hospital not far from home. I kept busy.

When our orders arrived to go to the Philippines, my daughter and I flew to San Francisco. We spent a week with my aunt before departing from Travis AFB, California.

We arrived in the Philippines, September 9, 1960.

Thom met us at the airport on base and drove us to our new home. As we drove, Thom joked. He pointed to a house on stilts and said, "This is where we will be living." I said, "It doesn't matter, as long as we are with you." Then he continued past the house on stilts and turned into a driveway with a house enclosed by a fence.

Our house was located in a neighborhood called Mountain View. We had to cook with propane gas and didn't have air-conditioning, but we always had a breeze throughout the house. The humidity was so high that we had to burn light bulbs in the closet day and night to keep our clothes from getting mildewed. I didn't complain because this taught me to appreciate the United States and our conveniences at home.

One day when Collette was playing in the sandbox in our yard, I heard her screaming. I ran to see what was wrong. Our yard boy had jumped the fence and picked her up. He brought her into the house and immediately put her under running water in the bathroom shower. Fire ants had gotten all over her. We got rid of the sandbox after that.

It was great to have a yard boy and house girl. Since the humidity was very high, I couldn't do much housework without getting sick from the heat.

Thom was still suffering from fatigue. He had to sleep during his lunchtime because he was forever tired. We now know that this is a major symptom of lupus, but at the time, we didn't know what was wrong with him. I continued to pray for his health.

In 1961, I became pregnant again, and our son, Keith, was born on August 25 at Clark AFB.

The birth of his son did not alleviate Thom's exhaustion. No matter how much sleep he got, he was still tired. The doctors continued to say that they didn't know what was wrong.

The poor guy continued having alopecia, sores in his mouth, and a constant tiredness—yet still no diagnosis.

I could understand why people thought Thomas was faking and not really ill. Sometimes even I would forget, because he looked good. He would not complain. He was just tired all the time, and each time he visited a doctor he had something different bothering him.

While Thom served his country in the Philippines, I made the best of it by attending sewing classes. That helped me psychologically, and I learned how to make patterns to sew clothes for the family.

I also taught Sunday school, volunteered with the squadron wives at schools we had adopted, and played bingo from time to time.

Oh, I almost forgot—if you like Filipino food, you will be interested to know that I became a top chef in making chicken or pork adobo, lumpia, and pancit.

Looking back, the weather in the Philippines reminds me of the weather in Florida, with its humidity, rainy seasons, typhoons, and hurricanes—plus lots of sunshine.

6

PENNSYLVANIA DUTCH AREA

Thom finished his tour in the Philippines in October 1961, and then we were stationed at Olmsted AFB, in Middletown, Pennsylvania. There I learned how to bank a fire, buy the right kind of coal, and keep the house clean of soot after the coal had burned.

In 1962, Thom was sent to Chanute AFB, in Illinois, for training, and he became very ill again.

When I learned that Thom was sick, I drove from Pennsylvania to Chanute AFB to be with him, traveling with two children who were ten months old and four years old. I would stop along the way to feed the kids, gas up, rest, and eat, and then I would start driving again.

One night, I drove until I found a motel located in a mobile home complex in West Virginia. I awoke in the middle of the night and felt the urge to get up and continue driving. I put both kids in the car in their pajamas and followed a bulldozer out of the area until the sun came up. Later, I passed the bulldozer and headed for Chanute AFB. When I arrived in Illinois, the headlines in the paper said that the area where I had stopped for the night was snowed in.

I continually praise the Lord for giving me the insight that we needed to continue our journey when we did, before the snowstorm hit the area.

■ ■ ■

Thom had been admitted to the hospital before I arrived, but the doctors still did not know what was wrong. He was put on medication for depression and was able to graduate with his training class.

Then he returned to Pennsylvania.

While we were living in Middletown, we visited Hershey, Harrisburg, Carlisle, Philadelphia, and Lancaster, and we even went shopping at the Oneida and Revere Ware factories outside of Rome, New York.

The Amish countryside was beautiful. We passed tall trees, flowers, and horse-drawn buggies as we drove through it. People in most Amish areas did not use TV antennas. You could see the beautiful blue skies above. The Amish ladies made beautiful quilts, canned fruit, and jars of honey that we could purchase from them.

In 1964, Thom was assigned to the Philippines again, and the children and I remained in Pennsylvania. While we were looking for a place to stay in Harrisburg, the real estate agent took us to see a home after dark. When he opened the door, roaches scurried all over. He told us he didn't want the neighbors to know he was renting to us until we moved in. As you can imagine, we did not rent that place. Instead, we found a nice duplex that we could rent to own in Harrisburg.

One evening, after the kids and I had lived in our duplex for about a month, my neighbor called at two in the morning. She told me to call the police because someone was stealing my hubcaps. I turned the porch light on, and the thieves ran.

When the police came, they found that three of my hubcaps had been stolen, even though Thom had welded them on with steel guards. The police told me not to worry because the insurance company would pay to replace them.

The next day, while I was at a service station paying for gas, I overhead someone say that one of his hubcaps had been stolen. We talked and discovered that our cars had the same type of wire hubcaps, which had recently been introduced. We realized that the thieves now had a complete set.

I bought a new set of hubcaps, but I didn't put them on until the car was shipped to the Philippines.

I had some good times in Pennsylvania. I remember taking some neighbors' children to see the Beatles. This was out of my league, because the girls in the audience were screaming, crying, and shouting.

7

TYPHOON EXPERIENCE

While he was in the Philippines, Thom had to rest during lunchtime because he was still feeling extremely tired. It seemed he just could not get enough rest.

He told the doctors that his sister had lupus, but no one listened to him. I guess that at that time, many of the doctors did not know what lupus was. They thought Thom was trying to avoid working.

Thom was still working as an electrical technician on airplanes in the hot sun while in the Philippines. He struggled to continue to do his job because he knew he had to take care of his family. He went to work sick many days. I cannot emphasize enough how exhausted he always was. He just could not get enough sleep.

Thom said that he was not afraid to die, but he wanted to know why he felt so bad. All the doctors he saw told him he needed to rest and not be stressed. Despite all the tests they gave him, they could not diagnose his problem.

He kept saying, "My sister Marion has lupus. Why don't they check me for lupus?" He slept a lot, and he often didn't like going places because he was always tired, in pain, or just not feeling good. I kept praying that things would get better for him.

■ ■ ■

After the kids and I joined Thom in the Philippines, we went to Manila, Baguio, Sangely Point, and Subic Bay. Baguio is a golf course in the mountains where many famous people go. To get there, we had to cross over a bridge that only one car could pass at a time. It looked like a rope crossing. I would close my eyes and pray. As I look back to that time, I remember it as a beautiful area, surrounded by mountains.

We visited a famous wall in Manila where the Japanese held the Filipinos captive. You could see where the prisoners had tried to dig through the cement to get out of the enclosure.

I have learned to appreciate my freedom and to try to help others understand that our freedom comes at a price.

■ ■ ■

A typhoon came through one year, and I will never forget it. Our home did not have glass windows, so the rain came through the window slats. I placed towels all around the floor to soak up the water, but it was useless. Thom said we should wait until the storm went through, because water would continue to come in until the wind and rain died down.

The electricity went out for three weeks, and many people lost all their food. I felt blessed because I did not have much in our freezer. It was just before payday, and I had not gone to the commissary. The base employees came by with ice for those who needed it so that their food would not spoil.

As I said before, all members of a family sacrifice in the military when they follow their loved ones. We have to leave family and friends behind. As it says in the Bible,

> Leave mother and father and cleave to your wife [husband]. (Genesis 2:24)

We could not drink the water in Angeles, the city where we lived. We were provided with large plastic bottles to fill with water on base for drinking and for cooking food. Our veggies had to be soaked in bleach and water to protect us from parasites and germs. We had to get used to the milk, which was reconstituted whole milk, and the carabao steaks and rations laws. Praise God, I had no trouble adjusting, because I was with Thom, and material things did not matter.

We used to comment that every time we made a move, we had to buy new curtains because our old ones never fit the windows in the new home. But we had each other.

A year before we returned to the States, we moved to the base and into a mobile home. I was very happy to have air-conditioning again as well as a regular stove to cook on.

■ ■ ■

At Easter time, we learned that some of the Filipinos crucify themselves, or allow themselves to be nailed to the cross, during Holy Week. This is done after they pray for someone in their family to be healed. They even flog themselves so their family member will be healed.

Not all Filipinos believe in this ritual, but it is a fairly common practice throughout the Philippines. Some of the people who are nailed to the cross die from infection, exposure, or other factors. They hang on the cross as long as Jesus hung on the cross.

■ ■ ■

During our stay in the Philippines, we visited the Negrita village, which was located on the base, twice a week. The Negritas are the descendants of the original inhabitants of the Philippines and are small in stature.

They were very poor, so I brought them clothes and food. They would not accept anything without giving us something in return. I was very proud of our son, Keith, when he gave one of the Negrita boys the toy gun he had gotten for Christmas. Keith realized that they didn't have toys like American children, so he gave the boy his treasured gun. He still gives away his best items.

They gave me knives they had made, and I found out later that while we were living on base, they were protecting our home from thieves.

When we were leaving for the States, the chief brought me his personal bow and arrows, which he had used for hunting. The arrows had points that would pull your insides out if you pulled them forward. Thom made me a wall hanging out of the arrows, but unfortunately, the bow was lost during shipping.

Being active in the community helped me cope with Thom's illness. I found that helping others gave me peace and satisfaction with myself.

8

OUR ROME ASSIGNMENT

Our next assignment took us to Griffiss AFB, in Rome, New York. Thom worked on airplanes in the cold and heat, and he was still having problems that were not diagnosed. During this time, Thom became very depressed. He still did not know what was wrong with him. Because of his illness, he was very worried about his commission in the military. He didn't know whether he would be able to stay in and perform his duties.

During our assignment at Griffiss AFB, our daughter, who was eight years old, became very ill. She was diagnosed with strep throat and sent home from school to recuperate. That evening, while sitting at the dinner table, she had no control over her hands. Her food was flying all over the table and floor, and she was unable to sit still. I told her to stop throwing her food, and she said, "I can't help it."

Terrified, we rushed her to the emergency room, and she was admitted to the hospital. We watched helplessly for days as she became worse. Again, I called upon the Lord.

One evening, I was sitting by her bed in the hospital praying, and I heard a voice say, "Give her to me." It was as if someone was in the room with me, but I couldn't see anyone. I replied, "OK, Lord. You can take her or leave her here with us, whatever you wish."

A few minutes later, a nurse approached me and said, "If you want your daughter to live, you need to take her where she can get help."

9

GOD'S HAND AT WORK

The next day, I went to my job in Utica working for Oneida County. I told my supervisor that my daughter was very sick and that the doctors at the base hospital did not know what to do for her.

A few days later, while I was at work, Thom called to tell me that Collette and I were going to be flown by plane to a hospital at Andrews AFB, in Maryland, the following day. My job gave me leave with the understanding that I could return when Collette was better. I won't say it was a bed of roses, because I loved to work and be around people. But my first priority at that time was to be with my daughter. My grandmother (Big Mama) came from Kansas to stay with Thom and Keith while I was in Maryland.

Later, I found out that my supervisor had phoned the base hospital and told them to send Collette to a hospital in Syracuse, New York, that specialized in children's illnesses. The hospital commander on base decided to send us to Andrews AFB, in Maryland.

When we arrived at the Andrews AFB hospital, a nurse took one look and said, "My God, she has rheumatic chorea." It was attacking her arms, legs, and head, causing jerky movements. Earlier, she had had rheumatic fever, which had turned into rheumatic chorea.

Collette was put into a dark room, and she began to get better. I finally saw what had gone wrong in New York. There, my daughter had been watching TV in a brightly lit room. The light had been aggravating her problem.

But I don't blame anyone. I know that the doctors don't know everything, so we have to turn to Jesus for help in healing.

> Evening and morning, and at noon, will I pray and cry aloud: and he shall hear my voice. (Psalm 55:17)

It was a blessing to see Collette improving daily. Thankfully, too, I have been blessed with many nice friends.

Friends who had been stationed with us in the Philippines had invited me to stay with them. They also gave me a car to use as long as I was in Maryland. Also, a couple of friends drove down from Utica to take me out for my birthday. They took me to the Ford Theater, the White House, and other sightseeing places. They spent two days with me. We still stay in touch.

■ ■ ■

After one month in the hospital, Collette was able to return home to New York, where she spent a full year at home recovering. She had to be carried for four months until her legs started working again. A tutor came to the house for third-grade lessons. Nine years later, she graduated from high school six months ahead of her class.

Once Collette was well enough, I returned to work for Oneida County as the supervisor for the mail room. One year later, Thom was assigned to Thailand.

10

TORNADO ALLEY

Thomas was stationed in Thailand in 1969, and the kids and I went to the "waiting wives" base in Salina, Kansas. This was a base for wives who were waiting for their spouses to return from overseas duty.

The first week after Thom left for his assignment, a tornado hit Salina. My grandmother called to see if we were OK. I told her it was just wind and rain, which is what the block leader told me when I asked whether it was a tornado. I should have known that it was a tornado. It was so dark that I couldn't see the house across the street.

My friend called me and told me she had heard a train going by. Her house was located in front of the train tracks, but I told her no one would be out in this kind of weather. It was just the wind and rain that she had heard.

The next morning when I got up and looked out the window, I saw sightseers driving by. I went outside and saw the damage the tornado had done. Our TV antenna was on the ground. Down the street, the tornado had turned the airplanes over. It had also gone through a trailer park. Fortunately, no one had been hurt.

Praise God, it went over the waiting wives housing area without hitting any of the homes. I thank God daily for taking care of us.

■ ■ ■

I sent Thom care packages every month with things he could not get in Thailand. It was a lot of fun shopping for the things he needed.

While he was in Thailand, Thom collapsed from exhaustion. He told me that he was exhausted and could not get enough rest. At the time, he was the only electrician in the area able to repair the planes. As usual, he had to sleep a lot to get more energy. Even though he was extremely tired, Thom continued to work on the airplanes.

I am sure the Lord was getting tired of my prayers, because every day I cried out to him for Thom's health and safety.

While Thom served our country, I worked at J. C. Penney, played softball, and made ceramics for family and friends. I also did a lot of sewing. In addition, I was able to spend time with my mother, grandmother, and great-aunt, which was one of the highlights of living in Kansas at that time.

After eleven months, Thom returned to the States. I met him in California, and then we went by train from California to New Mexico, where we stayed with our friends Loretta and Ed Mitchell. After our visit with them, we traveled to Topeka.

We picked up the kids, who had been staying with my grandmother and aunt. We then continued our journey to McGuire AFB, in Wrightstown, New Jersey.

11

JERSEY SHORE

After being on base for a year in New Jersey, Thomas was blessed to be able to retrain for the computer field.

I worked for six months as a cashier at a service station near our home. I later went to work at Fort Dix, processing GIs for discharge as they returned from Vietnam.

My supervisor from Fort Dix, his wife, and their friends took us on my first crabbing trip. I showed up dressed in my stockings and shorts, and everyone laughed at me. That was what I always wore, no matter where I went. I didn't know you waded in the water for crabs; and when they told me to throw the crab cage in, I did—rope and all. Thom had to wade into the water to get it.

Our son, Keith, was very young, and he didn't want to let any of the crabs get away. We told him that we wanted only the larger ones, but he was determined to catch some small ones.

After we returned to our friends' home, we had a crab feast. Keith wouldn't eat the small ones—he said they were too small.

■ ■ ■

My neighbor and some friends took me on my first trip to pick strawberries. Afterward, they had to share theirs with me because I had picked only a few berries. I had spent most of my time looking out for snakes.

Thom was still suffering with lots of pain, rashes, fevers, depression, lupus fog, exhaustion, and all of the frustration that had built up over the years. I suspected that he had lupus because I had seen how his sister had suffered. But the doctors were telling him that he was a hypochondriac. Every time he went to the doctor, something else was wrong with him. Little did they know that was how lupus attacks. It affects the liver, lungs, heart, kidneys, hair, and skin.

After spending two years at McGuire, we were assigned to Torrejon AFB, in Spain.

12

OLÉ!

One of our first meals in Spain was paella, a yellow rice dish that features shrimp, crab, and seasoning. The shrimp and crab are prepared whole and placed on top of the rice. I had to get used to seeing the eyes looking back at me on top of my food. It was delicious, though.

The following day, we went to a restaurant to practice our Spanish. We looked at the menu but didn't know what to order.

Thom asked for peppered steak in Spanish, and the waiter told him they didn't speak Spanish there—it was a French restaurant. When his peppered steak arrived, it was a steak with black pepper sprinkled on it.

We were hoping to find some tortillas, and we did, but they were not what we were used to or what we expected. A Spanish tortilla consists of eggs, onions, and potatoes and is prepared like an omelet in a skillet. Ours were delicious, but they were not the Mexican tortillas we thought we would be eating.

Spanish ladies are very private, but when you get to know them, they are very helpful. I made friends with some Spanish ladies who taught me how to shop for food daily. The food they prepared was always fresh. No one kept two weeks of food in the freezer, as we do in the States, and the refrigerators were very small. They brought me flowers, made a cake for my birthday, and took me around to meet their friends.

While we were in Spain, Thom's sister passed away with lupus. She was only thirty-nine years old, and she left behind five children ages eleven, ten, nine, eight, and six. We later found out that when women have lupus, giving birth causes the lupus to flare. Some women don't find out that they have lupus until they have a child.

Thom was still suffering with hair loss, depression, and pain. As his wife, I felt I had to stand by him because I had promised "till death do us part." I had to accept that Thom was sick, even though he never complained and did not look sick. However, I could see and feel his frustrations.

It has been a very interesting but challenging journey.

Car Accidents

One day Thom had a car accident on a slippery road. It was raining out. The car turned over three times. Praise the Lord, he had his seat belt on and was not hurt. While he was upside down in the car, he tried to knock the front window out. He had problems, though, because the window was shatterproof. A man stopped to help, but he couldn't kick the window out either.

Thom finally used a lot of force from inside the car and kicked the window out. The passerby helped Thom push the car back onto its wheels so he that could drive it home. It was a Seat, which is a Spanish car that looks like a Volkswagen but is even smaller.

When Thom walked in the door, I knew something was wrong because his uniform was dirty. He was in shock, but didn't know it. He asked me to take him to work after he changed clothes. While at work about an hour later, he called and asked me to take him home because he was shaking all over. It was delayed shock.

Some weeks later, I was in an accident. My car was hit in the rear and pushed into another car, which started a seven-car accident. The passenger in the car behind me was seriously injured when her head went through the windshield.

When you are an American in Spain and are involved in a car accident in which someone gets injured, you are usually sent back to the States. Everyone was wondering why I was not sent home.

In this case, the police happened to have a camera that had taken photos of the accident, and the photos showed I did not cause the accident. I was stopped, not moving, when the car hit me. The police had taken photos of my tire tracks in the road where I had stopped. This helped my case. It was clear that the car behind had pushed me into the car in front of me, and that action caused a chain reaction.

The driver of the car who hit me told the judge that I had a big American car, and the judge asked him, "What if it had been a Mack truck?"

It took one year to complete the court case. With the Lord's help, I won.

The judge asked me if I wanted anything for myself, and I said no. I asked only that my car be repaired. I spoke in Spanish, explaining what I wanted from the driver of the other car, and this behavior impressed the judge.

The doctor who hit me had to pay for the damages and buy the parts that were needed to complete the repairs on the car.

We had a second car, the Spanish Seat I mentioned before. One evening, we were going out for dinner and couldn't find the car. It was April Fools Day, and Thom thought at first that I had moved the car as a joke. We looked but did not find it. Finally, we asked a Spanish friend to go to the police station with us to interpret for us so that we could report that it had been stolen.

We went at six in the evening. If you have seen movies in which the policeman has a fan above him and is not rushing, you can imagine our situation. The policeman asked us to write down our mothers' and fathers' names and birth dates as well as other information. Our friend was laughing and making fun of the policeman in English while we were there. Our friend asked, "What do your parents have to do with a stolen car?" He laughed the whole time we were there. Eventually, all the paperwork was finished, but it was ten o'clock at night when we finally left the policeman's office.

They found the car four days later. Someone had taken it for a joyride and then had run out of gas. When Thom went to the police station to pick up the car, the policeman greeted him, saying in English, "Hello, Mr. Smith.

After Thom got home, he told our Spanish friend that the policeman could speak English and that he (our friend) was in trouble. Even a fool, when he holdeth his peace, is counted wise: and he that shutteth his lips is esteemed a man of understanding. (Proverbs 17:28)

■ ■ ■

We lived across from a bullring where we were able to go see a few bull-fights. Our son, Keith, would root loudly for the bull to win.

If a bull is aggressive and survives the fight, he is allowed to live. If the bull is slow and shows signs of weakness, he is killed. They drag the bull out of the ring to a designated place to be butchered. The meat is then taken to restaurants to serve.

Rewards

One of my most memorable times in Spain was being a secretary for the Torrejon middle and grade schools. I also taught a judo class to students in middle school.

The principal dedicated a yearbook to me and the janitor—that was a big surprise. It was the first yearbook that the Torrejon grade school had ever published.

Before we left Spain, my former supervisor from Fort Dix and his wife wrote us to ask if we would be the godparents of their daughter. We made arrangements to be in New Jersey for the christening when we returned to the States. Leslie is now a lawyer in New Jersey.

13

SACRAMENTO, HERE WE COME

After our four-year tour in Spain, we were assigned to Mather AFB, in Sacramento, California, where we would live for the next seventeen years. This was by far the longest that either of us lived in one place.

While we were in Sacramento, we bought our first home near the base. After living there for a year, we put it up for sale because we wanted to move to a larger home. Our real estate agent told us that it would be hard to sell because our price was too high and the light-rail tracks ran behind the house, but it sold the week the sale sign went up. When you have "faith as a grain of mustard seed," you can do anything.

During this time, Thom was again told by a doctor that he was a hypochondriac; the doctor told him that he should find someone else to treat him. So we found another doctor.

The second doctor discovered that Thom had water around his heart. A cardiologist performed a procedure that removed the water, but during this time, he also had a low-grade fever, alopecia, and pneumonia three times in less than six months. I know the Lord was looking out for Thom, because he would always recuperate and return to work. The Lord was not finished with Thom yet.

Many doctors in Sacramento were stymied about Thom's illness. They kept telling him that he was a hypochondriac and that they could do nothing for him. I was angry, but I couldn't do anything except pray that Thom found out what the problem was.

While we were living in Sacramento, Thom became very despondent after going to many doctors and not getting any results. One day, he went to a doctor and told him that he wanted to commit suicide.

The doctor called and asked me if we had guns in the house and told me that if we did, I should remove them. Thom was sent to the VA hospital in Palo Alto, California, and spent two weeks in treatment. The doctors told him that walking would relieve his symptoms. Thom followed their orders, but he still wasn't feeling well. That's when he decided he had to get out of there and find someone who could help him. He told them he was feeling better, so they released him that evening. He called to ask me to come pick him up because he was coming home.

Thom had always tried to keep on top of what was wrong with him, researching his symptoms and exploring ways to help himself.

That evening, we looked up the name of a psychologist and called for an appointment. The psychologist recommended that he see a psychiatrist; he said that he could give Thom biofeedback but that he felt Thom really needed medication.

The psychiatrist Thom later went to diagnosed him with deep depression and gave him a prescription for medication that he felt would help him. Fortunately, the medication helped Thom come out of the depression.

Thom now takes a small dose every day so he will not become as depressed as he was over the past years.

We have learned that to this day, Thom is experiencing post-traumatic stress disorder (PTSD). He served in Thailand for a year when the helicopters would fly in from Vietnam, and he would repair them. Thom worked on many helicopters that had blood and brains on the walls. He was affected by the gore and the stench, but he always did his job and continued repairing the helicopters for the missions.

■ ■ ■

At this time, our son, Keith, joined the army. Three years later, he was back with a diagnosis of schizophrenia and was admitted to the same VA hospital in Palo Alto where Thom had been a patient.

However, he escaped the hospital repeatedly. After escaping, he would call and say, "I am in a phone booth in San Francisco with my pajamas on, and I am cold."

Each time, I would call my brother to go get him and take him back to the hospital. Keith would always try to run home, but he couldn't get far because he didn't have money.

We have had to deal with his illness for the past thirty-six years. He doesn't trust anyone except his family members, and there are times when he doesn't trust us. It has been very difficult, but prayer has been my help and my strength, and it keeps me going daily.

■ ■ ■

I continued to work throughout this period. I worked for the US Army Corps of Engineers, a foreign exchange student organization, the Civil Air Patrol, and the Social Security Administration. I also did maintenance work as a forklift operator and worked at McClellan AFB, Mather AFB, and the Sacramento Army Depot. It was very rewarding, and I learned that you can do anything you put your mind to.

I also volunteered for the Miss Sacramento, Little Miss Sacramento, and Miss Rancho Cordova pageants. I would meet with the young ladies and teach them how to wear makeup and walk, as well as how to dress for success on job interviews.

I was blessed to have a very good friend who coordinated all these pageants. When she was injured, she asked me to help her while she recuperated. She not only taught the girls good posture but also taught them how to carry themselves and be good citizens in the community. She did not stress beauty because she said that beauty is in the eyes of the beholder.

I served as president of the Miss Black Sacramento pageant, and it was a thrill to see the girls grow with their training. I felt so proud when one of our pageant participants made an appearance on ABC's *Good Morning Show*.

14

I SEE THE LIGHT

When Thom retired from the air force in 1977, he had a job lined up as a computer operator at Cable Data. He worked two nights, then he quit.

His next job, a civil service position, was at the army depot. He started as a supply clerk and then transitioned into a more lucrative position as a material expeditor. Just before quitting time one day, a forklift hit his instep and broke his foot. We had been scheduled to go out dancing that night with people who celebrated their September birthdays together.

After the doctor placed a cast on Thom's foot, he told Thom not to go dancing; he knew the cement would need more than a few hours to dry. But he said he knew Thom would be a fool and go dancing anyway, so he would be waiting for him the next day. Thom went dancing that night, and he was the first patient the doctor saw the next morning.

Thom attended Bauder College while he was working at the army depot, and he graduated with honors with an associate degree in business management and marketing; however, he never worked a day in the field. He found that the army depot had more opportunities and benefits.

He had been looking for a position in electronics, and he finally obtained one. That position took him to a position that he really liked working with lasers, night vision, electronic repair, and IFF (identification, friend or foe) equipment.

When we learned that the depot was closing, Thom became very stressed out. He told me that he was praying for the Lord to take him out of the rat race of looking for a job. He said that he would go anywhere he was sent.

We put our house up for sale in case we had to relocate to another city, and it sold in two weeks.

We were asked by friends why we sold our house.

We told them we were not sure if Thom would be working in the Sacramento area, so we wanted to be ready for anything.

God's Country: Palmdale/Lancaster, California

We had once gone to the Palmdale/Lancaster area for a training meeting in cosmetics. When we left that area after the meeting, Thom said, "Who would ever want to live in this godforsaken land?"

Guess where the Lord sent us?

Thom's prayers were answered by an offer of a job at Edwards AFB in the Palmdale-Lancaster area.

We went by plane to Palmdale and looked for a home. Before leaving the area, we were blessed to find a home that was in foreclosure. Our real estate agent advised us that it might take a month before the bank closed the bids, but when we returned home a few days later, there was a message from our real estate agent saying that we were the proud owners of a new home.

I had stepped out in faith without a job in order to follow Thom. Then I was blessed with an offer of a job: I was able to transfer from the Sacramento Army Corps of Engineers to a similar position at the air force base in Palmdale.

Before we left for Palmdale, we found a church where we could worship.

> Pastor Ned of the Desert Winds Community Church was
> a friend of ours from Citrus Heights, California. He was
> the former choir director of the church we had attended
> when we lived in Sacramento.

15

MOJAVE DESERT

We left Sacramento after having lived there for seventeen years and moved to Palmdale, California, looking forward to a new adventure.

Thom's job in Palmdale was the best in his civilian career.

His office was in the high desert. Every morning when entering the building, he had to watch out for rattlesnakes that came inside looking for rats.

There were also plenty of ravens about. One day, the shop was having a party, and one of Thom's coworkers, Larry, brought corn wrapped up in tin foil. He left the corn in the back of the truck and went inside, and as he stood inside talking to the other people at the party, he saw pieces of tin foil raining past the window. Larry said, "Oh, my goodness." They all ran out and found ravens on the roof eating the corn.

Another time, Thom called me to his office on the hill to watch the shuttle land. My first sighting of the shuttle coming down behind the sun brought tears to my eyes.

■ ■ ■

In Palmdale, Thom went to many doctors, but they could not give him a diagnosis.

Finally, after we had lived in Palmdale for a year, Thom went to a dermatologist for help with his hair loss. The dermatologist did blood work and ran tests, and then he informed Thom that he had lupus.

He gave Thom a prescription for Plaquenil, hoping that would work for him. Thom was blessed to be one of the people that Plaquenil helps.

We were so happy to have a diagnosis that we didn't even care what the outcome would be. We were just glad to know that there was a name for his problem. It was such a relief to find out that Thom was not a hypochondriac.

During this time, Thom developed retractable drumsticks for drummers to take with them wherever they went so that they could practice drumming. They are convenient to carry, and they can be kept in shirt pockets; however, they cannot be used to play on drums because they are made of steel. We went to a few shows to advertise them, but Thom was not up to going to too many.

I started a cosmetics company called Brisa, and for a while, I was showing my products at shows and signing people up to sell them for me. But I sold all my products so I could spend more time taking care of Thom.

■ ■ ■

Thom had one of his bad lupus flares in Palmdale right after his diagnosis. He was not hospitalized, but he spent two months at home. He was having problems breathing and getting around the house. He couldn't even walk to the refrigerator or the bathroom without his blood pressure going up to two hundred. He had to crawl to the bathroom or kitchen when he had to use the bathroom or get something to eat or drink. I worked on the same base as Thom, fortunately, so I was able to share my sick leave so that he could continue receiving pay while he stayed at home.

Thom has always been a very good patient and never complains. I could see that his main concern was taking care of his family. I helped by working so that he would not have to work two jobs.

I thank God daily for allowing me to have a soft voice and a sense of compassion for others. I used to feel bad because I couldn't talk loudly—but thank God, I don't feel bad about it now. My soft voice has helped keep my son calm.

After Thom's diagnosis, and once he was feeling better, we joined a lupus support group in Palmdale/Lancaster. I saw a big change in Thom when he saw that he was not alone with lupus.

I learned more about lupus and how other people coped with it. I saw that everyone with lupus is not the same. You can have a room full of people with lupus, and each one could have a different complaint at that time. I also found that the sun, medication, stress—and possibly family genes—cause lupus. I saw that some of the people were affected by taking heavy doses of steroids for a long time, and they would swell up from the medication.

■ ■ ■

Our yard was so big that it took Thom two days to mow the front and back. He also had to take care of one hundred and fifty trees. We had to hire a young man to do the work for us because Thom was not able to do it.

Thom wanted to sell the house, but he was afraid at first to tell me, since he knew that I loved the house so much. But when he approached me about selling it, I agreed that we should. I knew that he couldn't continue doing the work. I have never been in love with any material thing that I couldn't give up.

Two months later, the house sold for our asking price. The next month, housing prices dropped, and I knew that it had been the Lord guiding us to sell our home.

We moved into a townhouse where I met a new neighbor who told me she had just been diagnosed with lupus. She was very distraught. I shared with her what I knew about the disease. I asked her about her symptoms, and she said that they had appeared out of the blue. She also told me that she had breast implants, so I told her to have them checked. I had read an article about implants being a problem for some women. If the implants broke or leaked, they could cause illnesses.

She went to her doctors, and they found that one of the implants had caused her problems. When they removed the implants from her body, her symptoms of lupus went away.

16

YOU DON'T LOOK SICK

People with lupus feel frustrated because they want to work but cannot perform. They don't look like they are ill, but their bodies are attacking their organs. They are often docked for being late or for being unable to perform their duties because many supervisors do not understand that they are sick.

The illness and its wide range of symptoms keep people with lupus from being able to live a normal life. They also have to wait a long time to get social security benefits. In addition, some patients don't have the support of their spouses. Because people with lupus don't look sick, their spouses may feel that they are faking illness.

Very few doctors understand the symptoms of lupus, and many doctors are unable to diagnose it. Lupus is very difficult to diagnose if you don't have insight into its symptoms. Furthermore, some people with lupus can also have overlapping diseases, including scleroderma and fibromyalgia. They are in terrible pain at times and cannot get out of bed.

Thom was always feeling bad. He worried that he would not be able to work and support us, but he persevered and fought the odds so that he could do his job.

17

GATOR TERRITORY

In May 1999, Thom retired from civil service, and we moved to Clearwater, Florida. Thom was going through another bad lupus flare during our move.

In September 1999, I took Thom to the VA in St. Petersburg. The doctor there was angry with him because he didn't have his medical records. He told Thom to come back in two weeks.

That evening, Thom was notified that his mom was very sick, but he was so ill that he couldn't think. The next day, we received a call to say she had died. I made arrangements for us to go by train to New Jersey from Florida.

In New Jersey, we made the arrangements for his mom's funeral. But the day before her wake, Thom asked me to take him to the emergency room at Elizabeth General Hospital because he couldn't take the pain and awful feelings any longer.

As soon as we arrived in the emergency room, they did various tests, including a blood test and X-rays. Thom's toe had turned black from a medication he had taken for pain. His oxygen was also very low, so they put him on oxygen and strong medications.

Thom told the doctor that his mom's wake was the next day and her funeral was the following day. He said that he had to leave the hospital.

But they told him that he wasn't going anywhere; he was too ill to leave the hospital.

Thom was admitted to the same hospital his mom had died in earlier that week.

Thom told me he believed that his mom had died so that he could go to Elizabeth, New Jersey, to get treatment from doctors who knew about lupus. He spent two weeks in the hospital.

I returned to Florida to get the car. I put the car on the train in Sanford and then got off the train in Virginia and drove north to New Jersey.

■ ■ ■

When we returned to Orlando, we contacted the Winter Park/Orlando lupus support group, and they supplied us with doctors' names and phone numbers.

We found Dr. Sheikh, whom Thom still sees after fifteen years of treatment. The doctor told me not to worry about Thom because he was in good hands. The doctor didn't even want to see the tests done by other doctors. He said that he would run his own tests, and then he would make his own decisions.

He put Thom on chemo and prednisone. Thom came out of his flare four months later. When he felt a little better, we attended the lupus support group meetings in Winter Park/Orlando. Again, I saw a change for the better in Thom when he saw that he was not alone and that others were suffering like him. That was the beginning of Thom's fight to learn more about lupus and share with others.

We participated for about three years in the Winter Park/Orlando group. Then Thom and I started a support group in Clermont, Florida.

During a good patch, we went to work for Universal Studios. We went for two days of training and on the third day, we went to work on the turnstiles. I told Thom I did not want to work anymore because it was too hot and because I had to rush all the time. The tickets would not work if they were bent or chewed on. People were standing in line angry and irritated because they wanted to get into the park.

He said, "You can do it."

The next morning at 2:00 a.m., Thom woke and said, "Heck no, I'm not going back to work." We went back that morning and turned our uniforms in.

Thom bought a device that allowed him to make a tent so that the covers would not touch his feet or legs while he slept. Anything that touched him caused severe pain.

> I will cover you all day long as you rest between My shoulders. (Deuteronomy 33:12)

18

HOPE

Our group in Clermont was not one in which the participants felt sorry for each other. We shared updated information, shared how everyone felt, heard from various speakers, and enjoyed our parties. Every year, we had a Christmas party during which we played the white elephant game and had a potluck with good food. People came whether they were in pain or not.

I could see the hope, excitement, and love in our group.

We prayed and thanked the Lord for allowing us to be with the group each time we met.

I also thank God for being able to see and better understand what lupus is doing to people. I pray that more doctors will become aware of the symptoms of lupus so that they will be able to diagnose people with lupus before they suffer for many years without knowing what they are suffering from.

People with lupus are not trying to get out of work.

They get tired easily because the disease is attacking their heart, muscles, legs, kidneys, hair, nervous system, and skin. They have lupus rashes. When people see the rashes, they often worry that it is a disease that they can catch. They don't understand the disease or its symptoms.

Believe me, it is an autoimmune disease that doctors need to be more knowledgeable about in order to help alleviate the pain and suffering it causes.

We all have to die, but some of us suffer most of our lives. Sadly, three of our members died. Each of them fought a long battle but left a legacy of love and hope.

One very troubling memory I have is of someone who couldn't work long hours whose dad told him he was just lazy and not sick.

To prove to his dad that he was not lazy, he went to work when he was ill. He died two weeks later from lupus complications.

We have to be aware that there can be problems that are unseen. Everyone says, "You don't look ill, you look good," but the problems are within.

We have to be aware that there are diseases that attack the autoimmune system that do not show on the outside all the time.

19

NEVER GIVE UP

In December 2015, we went on vacation to Tampa. Thom had been in remission for three years. While we were away, he developed a low-grade fever, sores in his mouth, and lupus fog, and he was just not feeling well. But he didn't want to disappoint me, so we continued our vacation. While he slept, I went shopping, sightseeing, and walking. He didn't want to go to a doctor because he knew he was only having a slight flare. He usually just coped with those until it was over.

In January 2016, he had another lupus flare that he is still coping with. (I am writing this in September 2016.) He went to the emergency room, thinking that the doctors would give him a shot for his lupus rash. One doctor told him that he had herpes, and another doctor told him he had shingles. I told them it was lupus, but they didn't believe me. Thom jokingly asked the doctor how many marriages had he broken up by telling the spouse that their loved one had herpes.

After that, I took Thom to his rheumatologist, Dr. Sheikh, and he agreed that it was a lupus flare. He gave Thom a shot for his rash and pain. He also prescribed ten milligrams of prednisone. This helped the lupus rash, but Thom was still in pain. So they took two MRIs and found that he had a torn rotator cuff with spurs as well as arthritis in his neck with pinched nerves. He went to three doctors to finally be cleared to have three epidurals. Praise God, he has no more pain in his neck after the third epidural.

Later, he had a sciatica attack, and he had to have three epidurals in both sides of his hip.

Thom is still suffering with back pain, but he is reading up on it and trying all types of contraptions to ease the pain. He never stops researching in an effort to get relief with or without medication.

Recently, Thom wanted to go to Delaware to visit our goddaughter's family. He was in pain but told me that even if I had to drag him up the train steps, he was still going.

We did go, and we had a wonderful time with our goddaughter and her family.

We stayed with Leroy and Linda in New Jersey. While there, we attended church, shopped, and enjoyed a crab feast that Leroy prepared. They were also kind enough to drive us to Columbia, Maryland, to see Cynthia and Hubert.

Leroy also drove us to Jackson to visit Thom's cousin, where we prayed for her health and well-being.

While we were on vacation, we had two crab feasts, and I went shopping every day. I also did a lot of walking, but one day I had to stop because the humidity was too much for me. It was a blessing not to have to drive everywhere, so I just relaxed and enjoyed everything.

The Lord has blessed us with very good friends, and we will never forget them.

Restrictions

For some reason, lupus patients often have to wait for years to receive medical support. Many doctors don't know what to look for and cannot make a correct diagnosis. Since we never know when the lupus will attack, we live from day to day. Usually we don't make long-range plans. We purchase travel insurance so we can use the reservations another time or get a refund if we cancel.

We no longer go on cruises or fly because of the risk of flu or lupus flares. Our past travels were in large crowds and resulted in Thom having a flare every Thanksgiving or Christmas for five years.

We have been on two cruises, but we didn't enjoy them. We didn't like having to rush to get back to the ship, and we didn't like going to tourist traps. What we enjoy most is going from city to city, shopping in different stores, looking the town over, and just relaxing. So we have decided to ride the train or drive wherever we want to go. With the Lord's help, we will thrive and be able to share our experiences with others.

No Cures

We understand that there is no cure for lupus and that the lupus flares can attack any time. These can cause kidney failure, heart attack, and problems with the eyes and with breathing. Lupus also affects the brain, and it can leave the person with lupus unable to walk; he or she can become wheelchair-bound. But no matter what happens, as long as the Lord allows me, I will be by Thom's side to support him in his illnesses.

The doctors do not know for sure whether lupus is hereditary, but I feel that it is in some cases. I see so many families with two or three members who have lupus while other family members have other autoimmune problems. In addition to his sister, Thom has a niece and cousin with lupus and other cousins with autoimmune diseases.

> For a just man falleth seven times, and riseth up again.
> (Proverbs 24:16)

There is now a medication especially for people with lupus. It is called Benlysta. It was approved by the Food and Drug Administration for the treatment of lupus on March 9, 2011.

20

ALZHEIMER'S AND LUPUS

In 2012, Thom was diagnosed with the beginning stages of Alzheimer's disease.

At first, when he showed symptoms of Alzheimer's, I was impatient with him. But now that I know what is going on, I have adjusted. I changed my attitude because I now understand what he is going through.

I am always on a roller coaster because we never know when Thom will have another lupus flare, but I have come to depend on the Lord for all my needs. My faith helps me to know that the Lord is always there. I try to be obedient to the word of God.

I used to be upset because I couldn't yell or speak loudly, but now I see my God-given gifts. I see that I love to organize and see that everything is working out for the good of everyone, and I see that I am meant to be calm and speak softly to others.

> I know that if we use our God-given gifts to the fullest, we
> will be rewarded with more than we can fathom.

Prayer helps me a lot, and now it is easier for me to accept that Thom needs my care still after fifty-nine years of marriage. God has shown me how to treat others with love.

Today I have given Thom's care to the Lord, because I cannot heal him or help him by worrying. But supporting Thom through his illnesses is a blessing to me. At one time, I wanted to be a police officer so that I could help others. Now the Lord allows me to be there to help Thom.

I see Thom handling his lupus and his Alzheimer's very well. He is very loving and helpful in whatever I do. He never gives up. He has faith in God and knows that without Him, he could not survive.

I thank God for the many years that He has given me with Thom. Our marriage was a God thing.

Through it all, I have grown stronger in my faith. When I find that outside things are clouding my vision, I turn my eyes back to Jesus. I do not watch the news because television clouds my vision. The Bible is my news—that never changes. It has good news that keeps me focused on the Lord.

Without my faith in Jesus Christ, I could not be where I am today. Join me in knowing the Lord for your salvation and peace of mind.

ACKNOWLEDGMENTS

Without the following people and groups, this book would not have been written: Thomas Smith Sr. and Lillie Bell Smith, Thom's mother and father; Marion Smith, Thom's sister, who died at the age of thirty-nine from complications of lupus, leaving behind five children under the age of twelve; and Thomas Smith Jr., my husband of fifty-nine years.

Special thanks go to the lupus support groups of Palmdale/Lancaster, California; Winter Park/Orlando, Florida; and Clermont, Florida.

Heartfelt thanks also go to friends: Pastor Ned and Wendy Beadel, Dr. Bill and Marilyn Bellavia, Pastor Ben and Beth Bond, Ryan and Dorothy Cochran, Ann and Earl Lee, Ken and Vicki Ley, Levi and Mary Merritt, Leroy and Linda McNair, Loretta and Ed Mitchell, and Vivian and Larry Van Cleave.

All scripture quoted in this book is taken from the Holy Bible, King James Version.

Twila McKay-Smith graduated from Topeka High School. She has worked in government for twenty-five years.

McKay-Smith has received many community awards for her work. She has also coordinated fashion shows and attended Barbizon Modeling School.

McKay-Smith lives with Thom, her husband of fifty-nine years, in Clermont, Florida.